How Summer Came to Canada

Pictures by
ELIZABETH CLEAVER
Retold by William Toye

Toronto   Oxford   New York
Oxford University Press

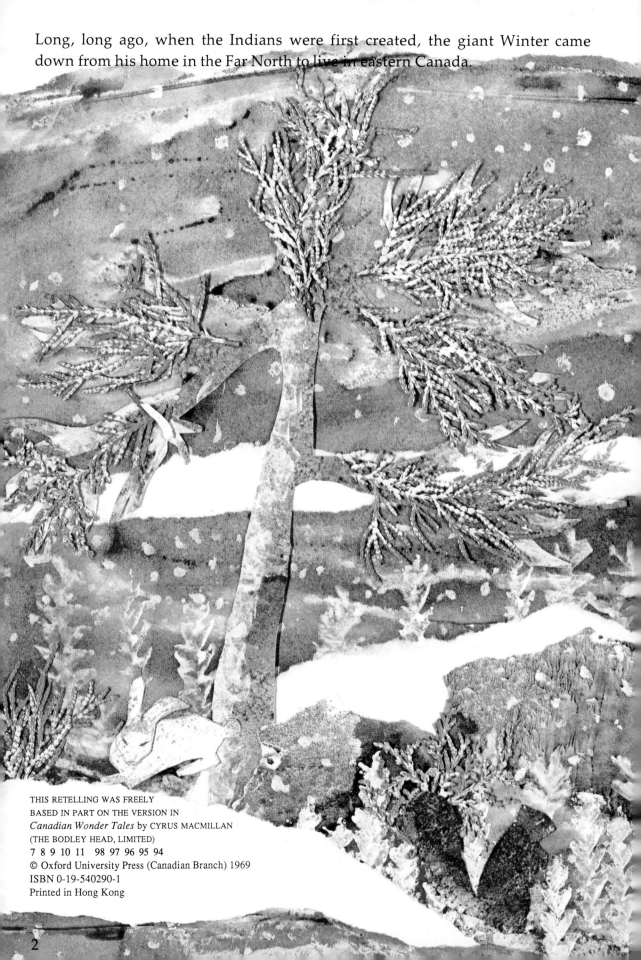

Long, long ago, when the Indians were first created, the giant Winter came down from his home in the Far North to live in eastern Canada.

THIS RETELLING WAS FREELY
BASED IN PART ON THE VERSION IN
Canadian Wonder Tales by CYRUS MACMILLAN
(THE BODLEY HEAD, LIMITED)
7 8 9 10 11 98 97 96 95 94
© Oxford University Press (Canadian Branch) 1969
ISBN 0-19-540290-1
Printed in Hong Kong

As he breathed on the trees and flowers and passed his icy hand over mountains and fields, all the once-green land became frozen and white.

3

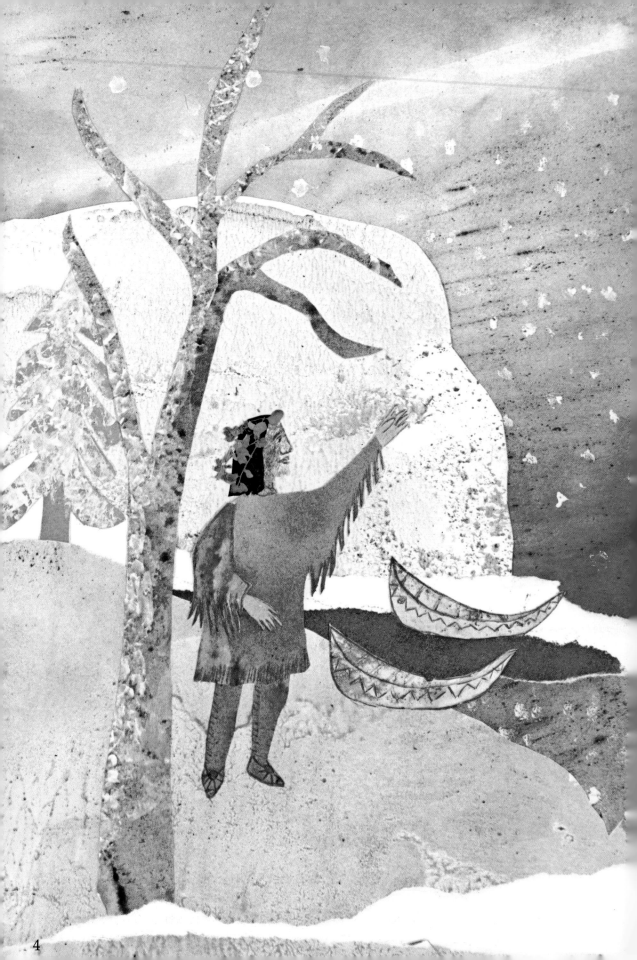

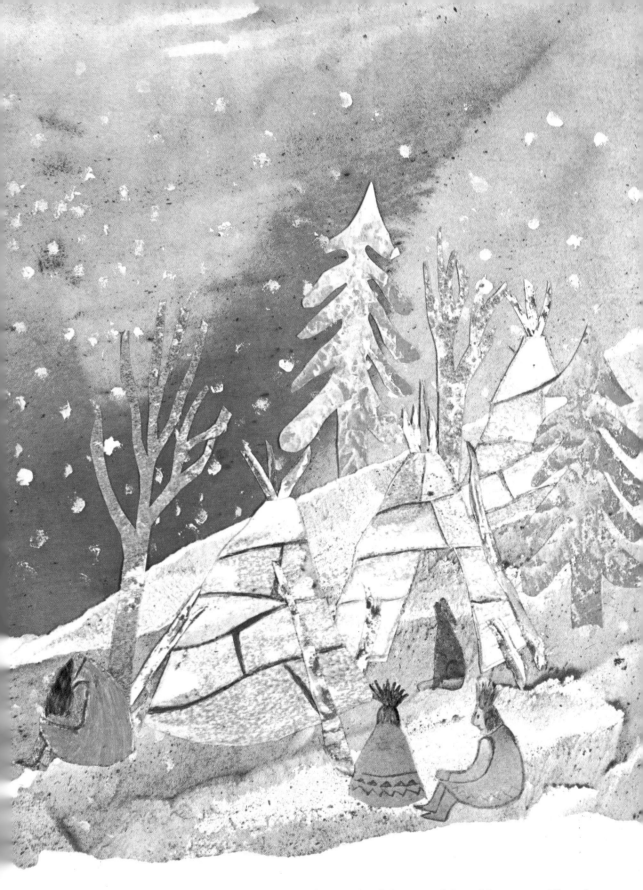

Nothing grew anywhere and the Indians died from cold and hunger. Glooskap, their lord and creator, decided to use his magic powers to send Winter away.

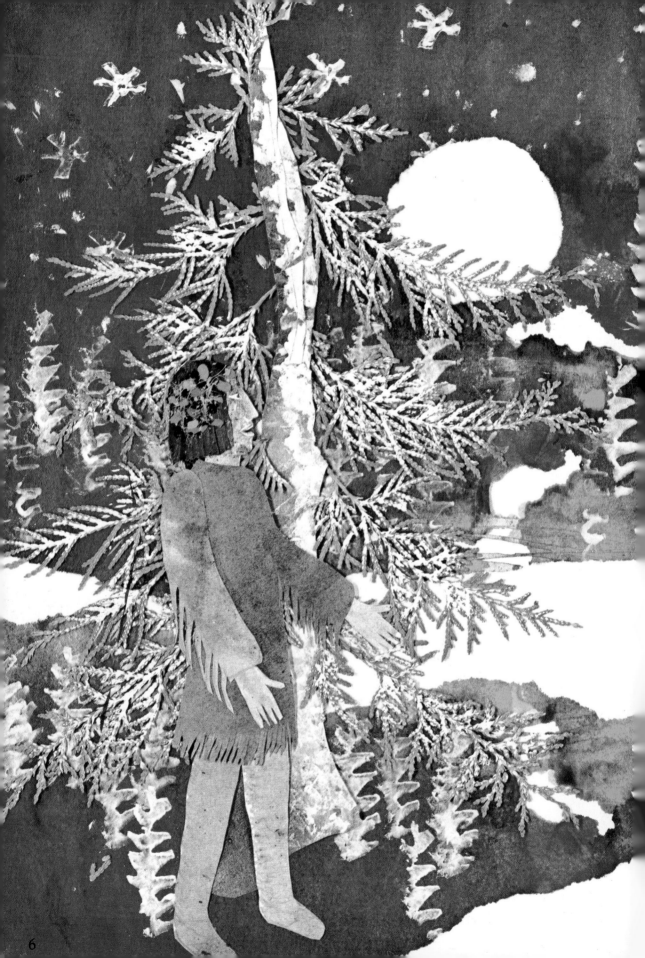

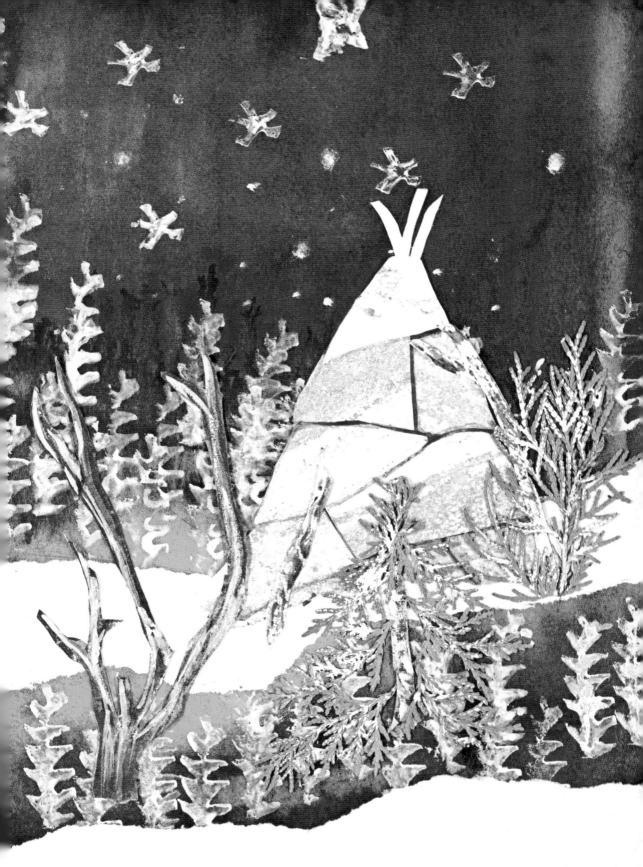

He went to the beautiful place where Winter lived. The giant's tent glistened white and cold in the rays of the moon. Above it the sky was filled with flashing, quivering lights and the stars shone like diamonds.

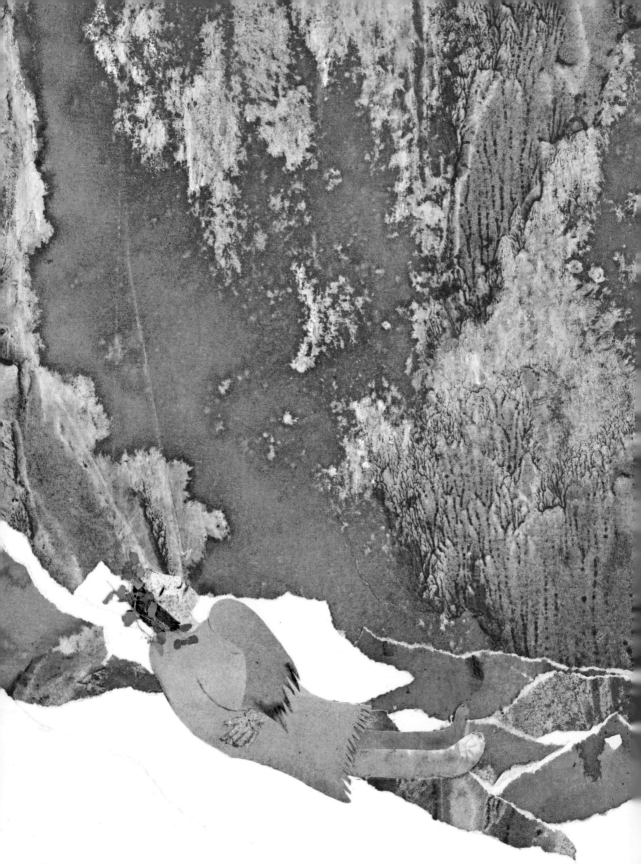

When Glooskap entered the tent, Winter made him welcome. But before Glooskap could use his magic powers to send Winter away, Winter cast a spell on him. He proceeded to tell Glooskap tales of ancient times when the whole

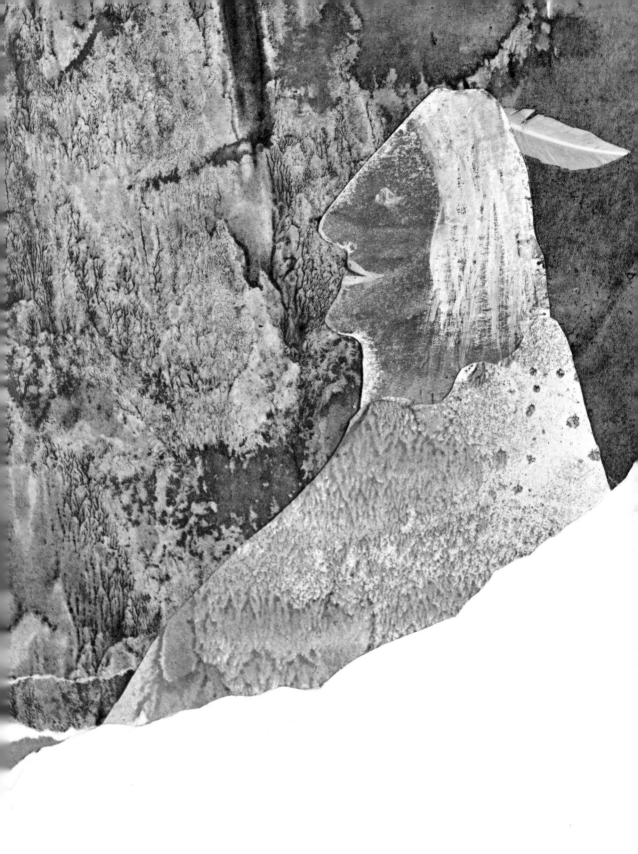

world was covered with ice and snow. Glooskap forgot the reason for his visit and felt a great longing to stay with Winter. He became drowsy. He fell into a deep sleep and had a dream.

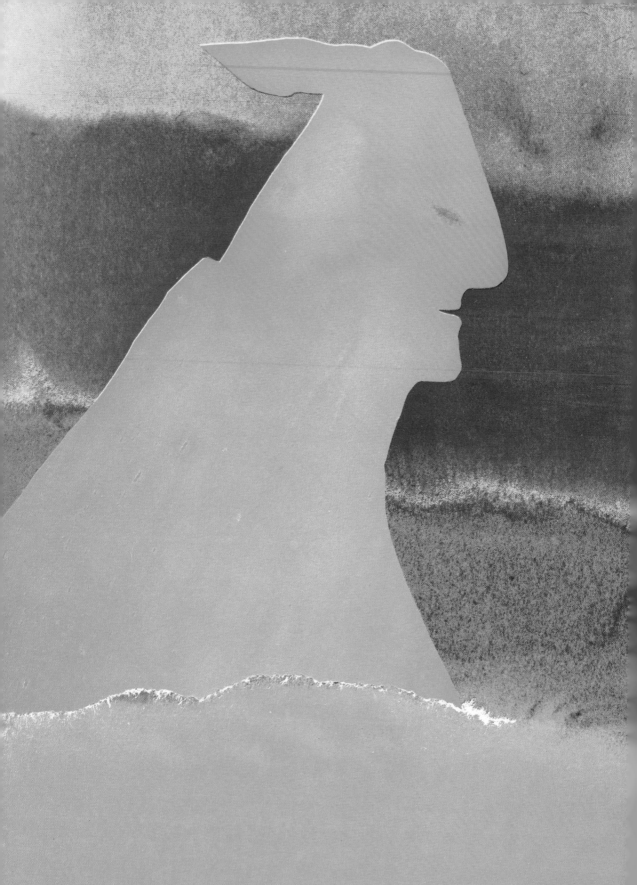

The giant Winter, looking cold and menacing, loomed over Glooskap in his dream.

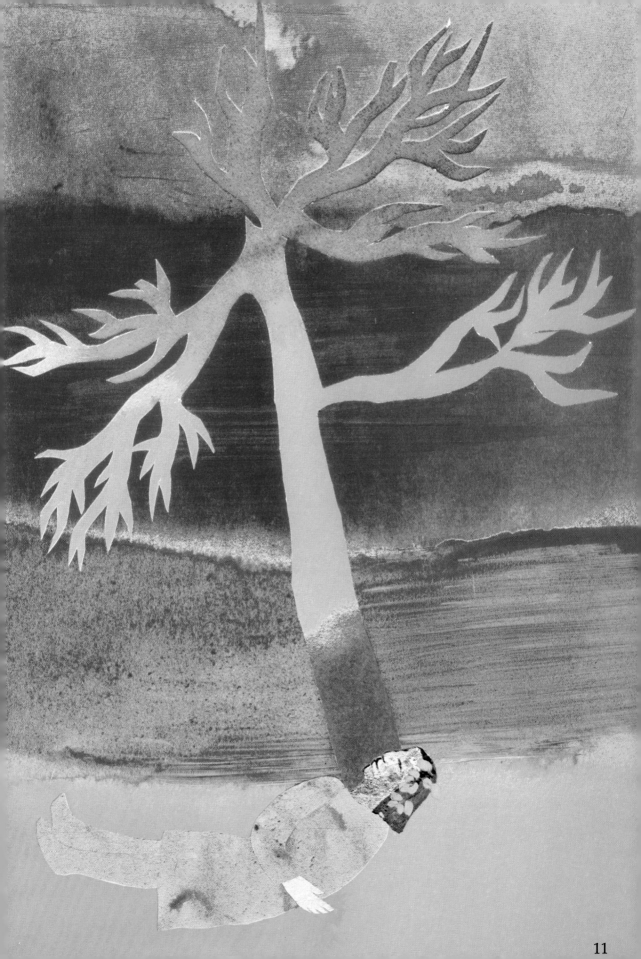

Then suddenly he grew smaller and smaller. The smaller he became the faster
the ice and snow melted, until they made raging torrents of water.

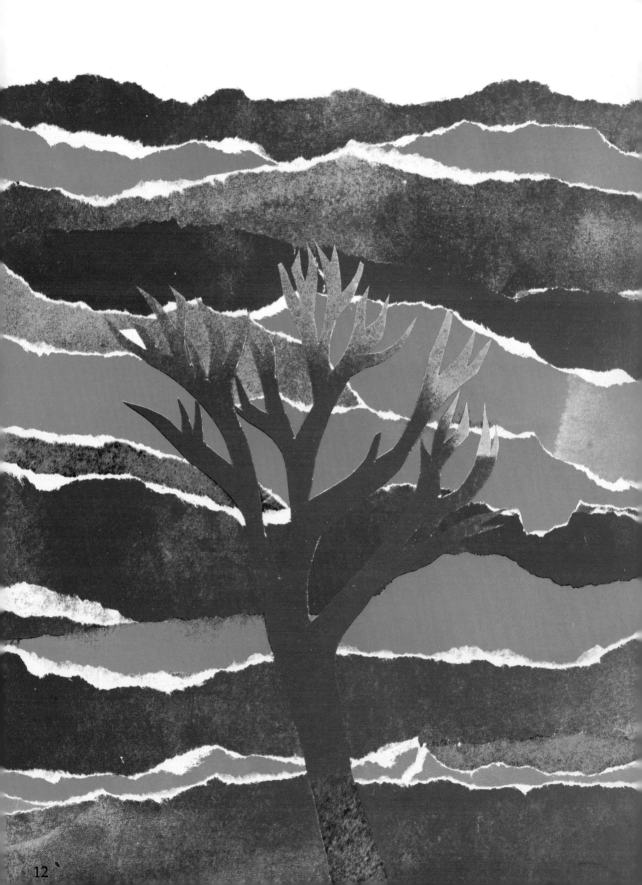

When Winter had all but disappeared and the land turned green again, the dream ended. For six months Glooskap slept like a bear.

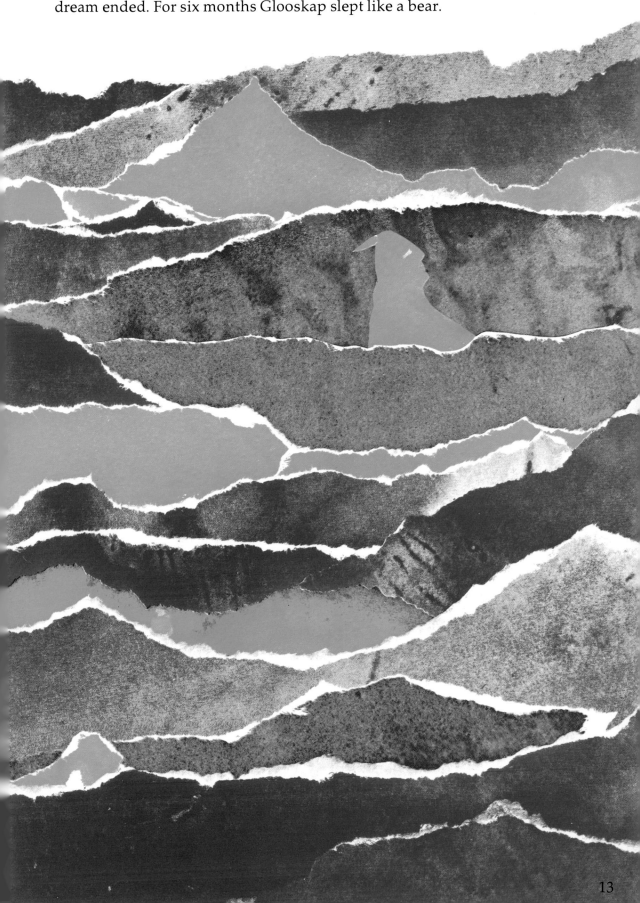

When Glooskap woke, his friend Loon appeared before him. "There is a land far away in the South," he said "where it is always warm. A Queen reigns there and her power is greater than the giant Winter's. Go to her and bring her here."

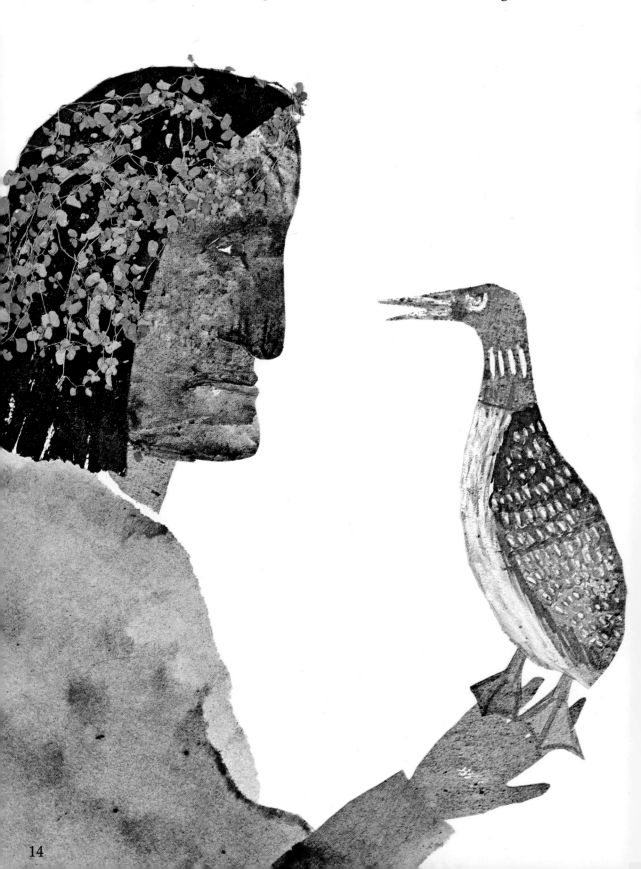

So Glooskap went to the ocean, many miles away, and called for Whale. He jumped on Whale's back and together they sped through the water for many days, until the ocean became warm and the air sweet with the fragrance of flowers and pines. When Glooskap looked into the clear green depths of the sea and saw white sand beneath him, he slipped off Whale's back and swam ashore.

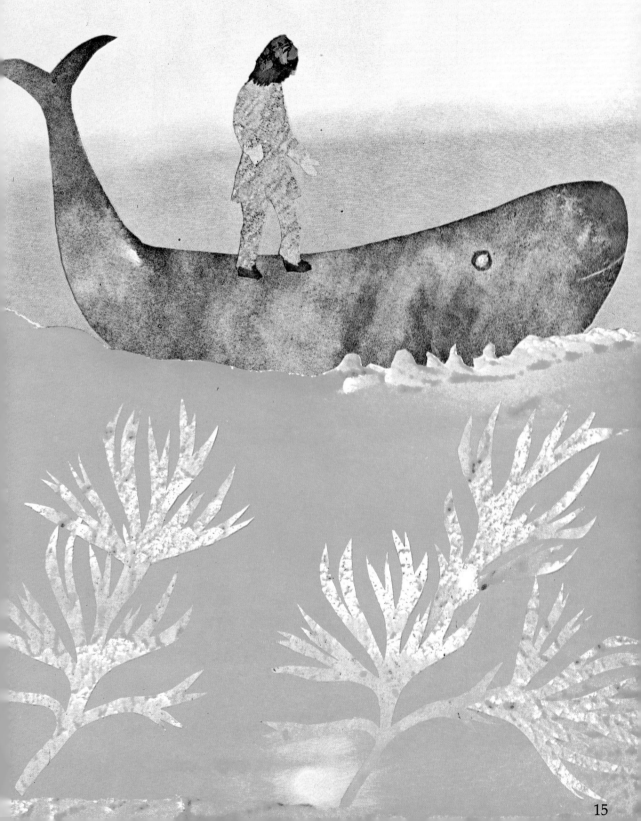

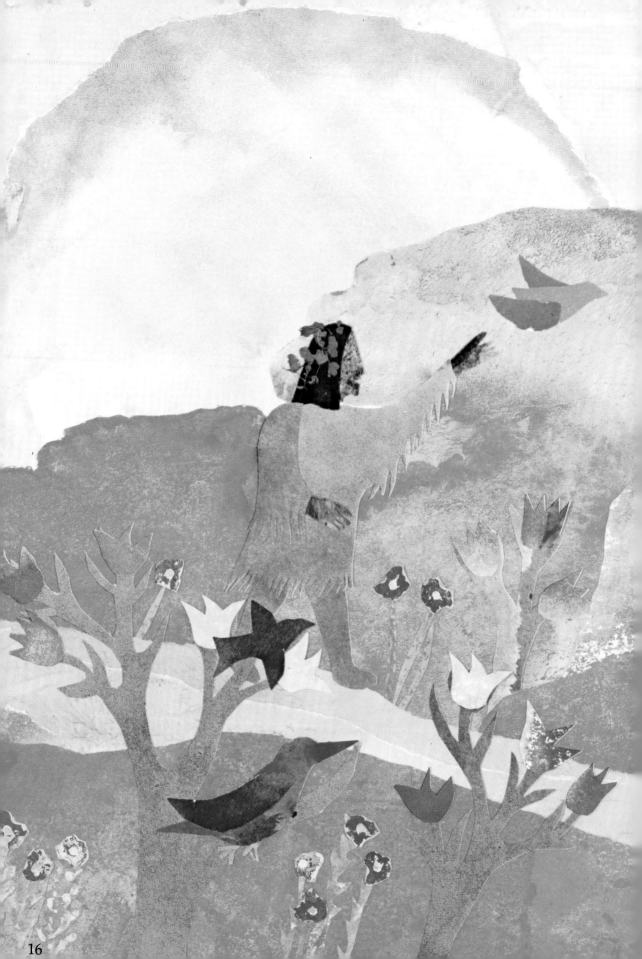

With great strides Glooskap walked far inland along a flower-lined road. Tulip trees grew on either side, birds of brilliant plumage sang in their branches, and wherever flowers or trees did not grow, the ground was covered with velvety grass.

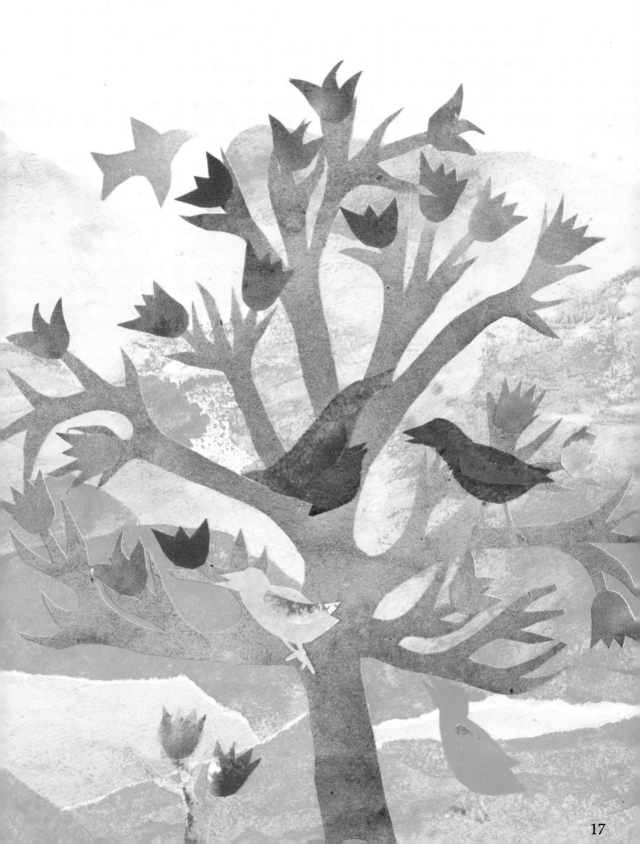

He came to a grove where he heard voices raised in song. He peered through the trees and saw four maidens singing and dancing in a Wilderness of Flowers. They held blossoms in their hands and circled around the fairest woman Glooskap had ever seen.

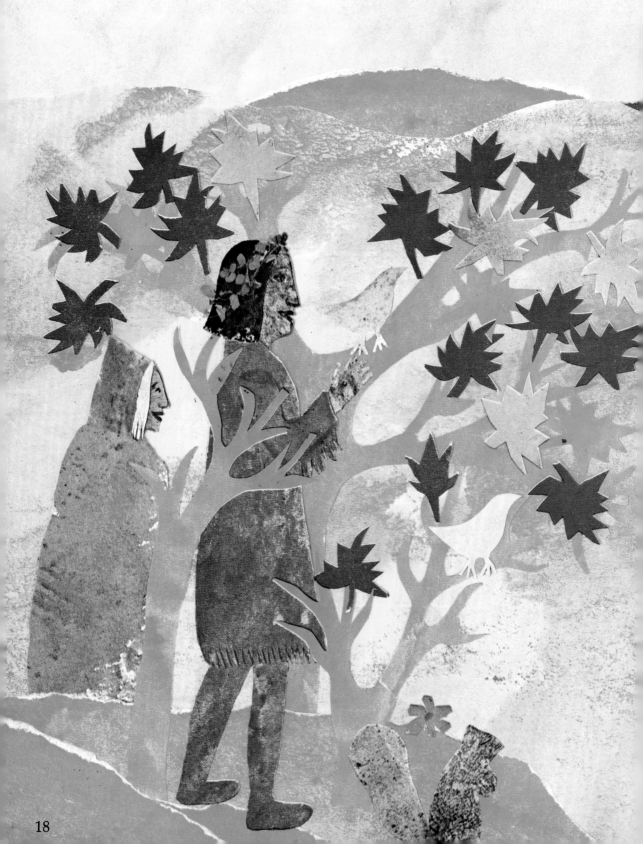

When he recovered from his surprise, Glooskap noticed that a little old woman stood beside him. "Who are these maidens?" he asked her. "The Fairies of Light and Sunshine and Flowers," the old woman answered. "They dance around their Queen. Her name is Summer."

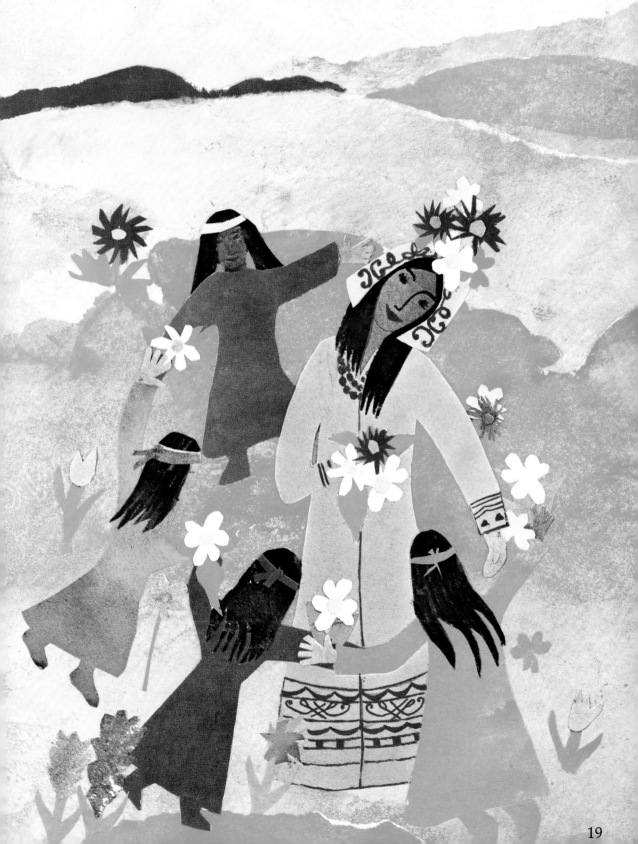

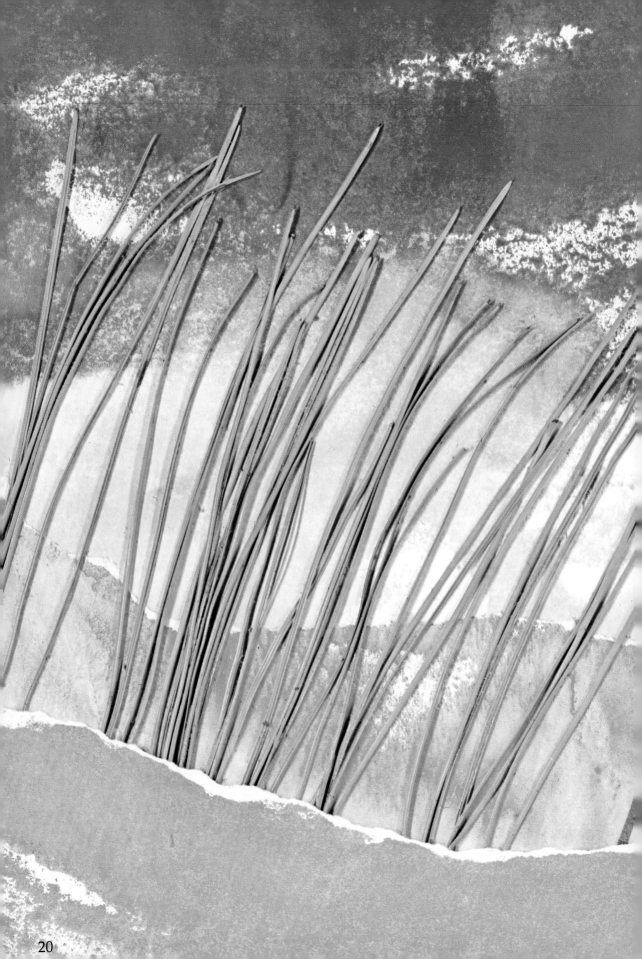

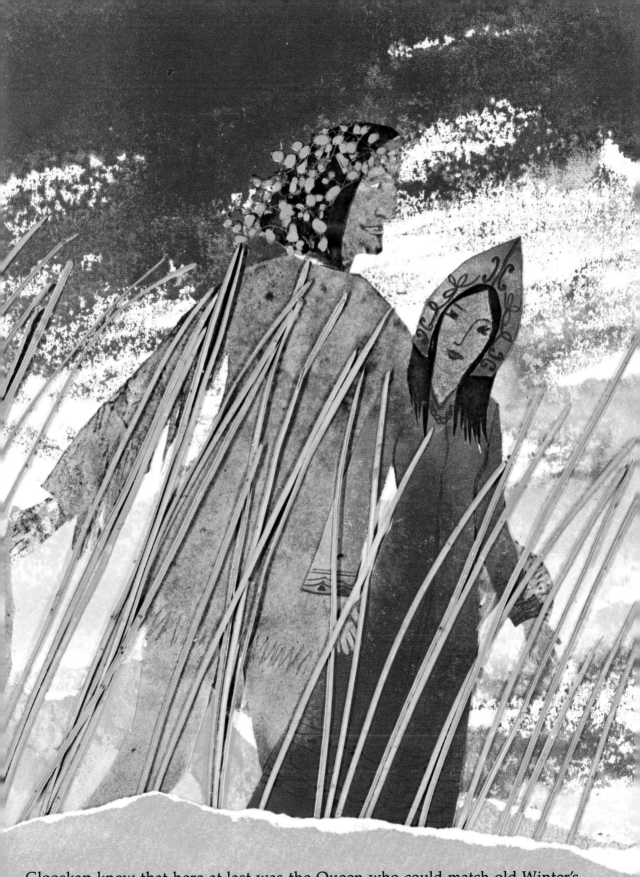

Glooskap knew that here at last was the Queen who could match old Winter's power. He sang a magic song. When the Queen heard it she willingly left her maidens and went to Glooskap. Unravelling behind him a slender cord of moosehide, he raced away with Summer.

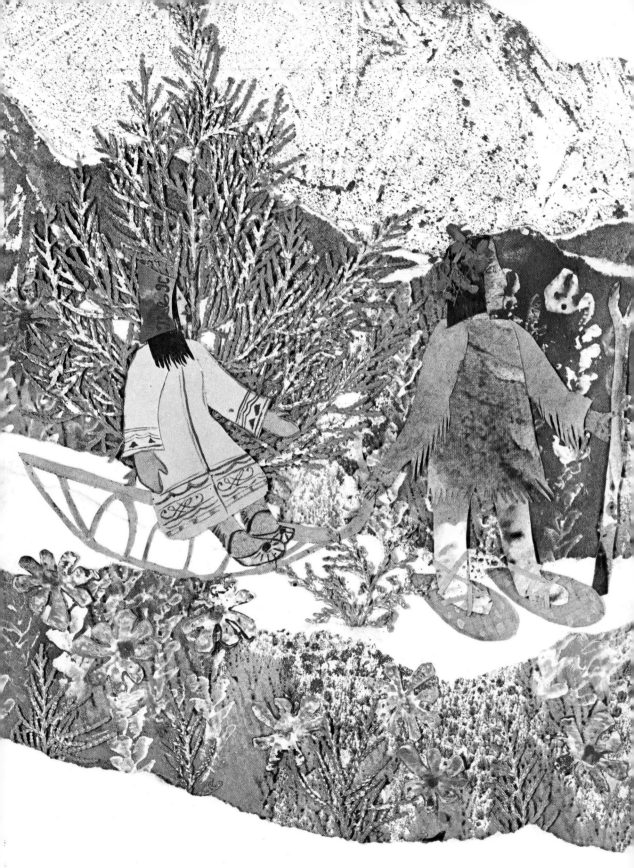

After many days Glooskap and Summer reached the Northland. The people were all asleep; the cold and lonely land was also asleep under Winter's spell.

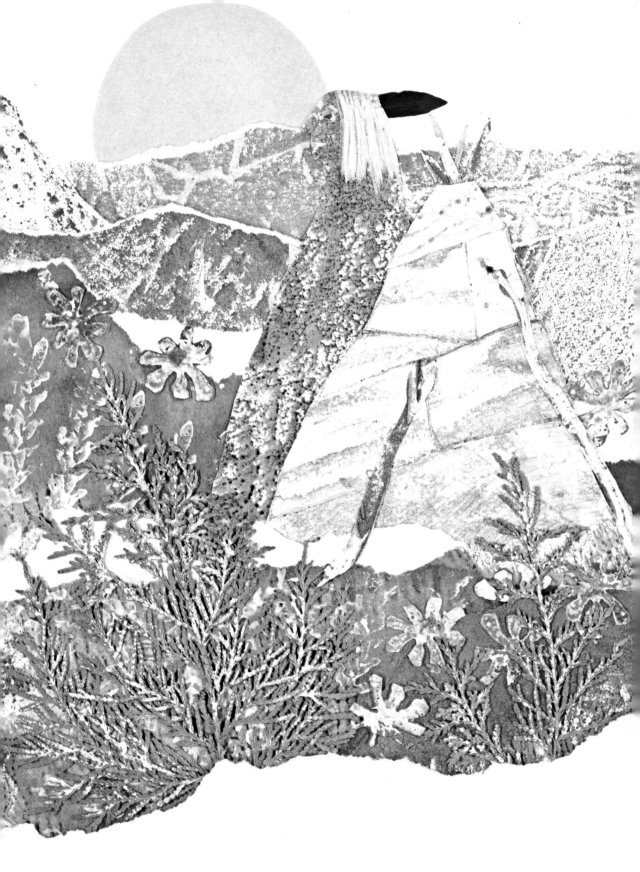

Winter's tent gleamed in the morning sun. The giant was overjoyed to see Glooskap again. He determined to keep him with him always, and Summer too, by casting his strongest spell.

But the power of Summer was changing the frozen land. Ice and snow were turning to water. New grass and leaves showed that the earth had returned to life.

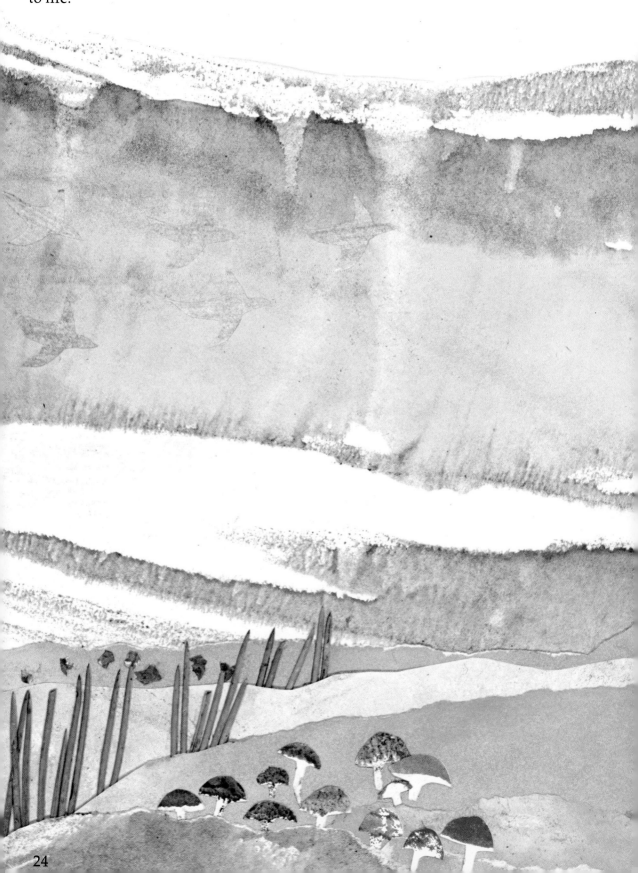

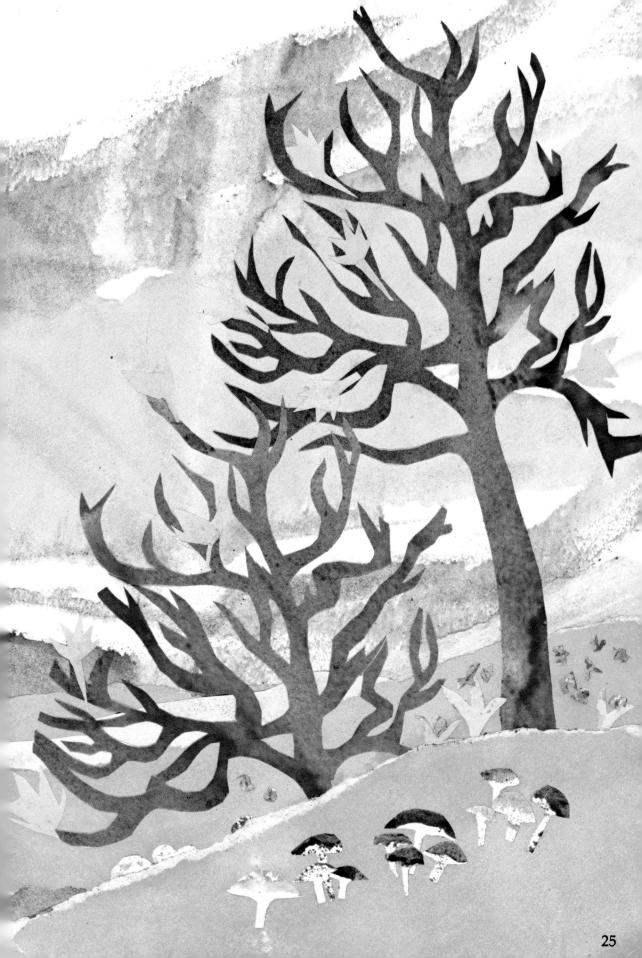

Even old Winter was melting away. He wept and his tears fell like cold rain on all the land. Summer took pity on him. "I love Glooskap's country and want to

stay," she said, "but we cannot live here together. Return to your home in the North for half the year. When you come back, I will never disturb you. But I will rule when you are away."

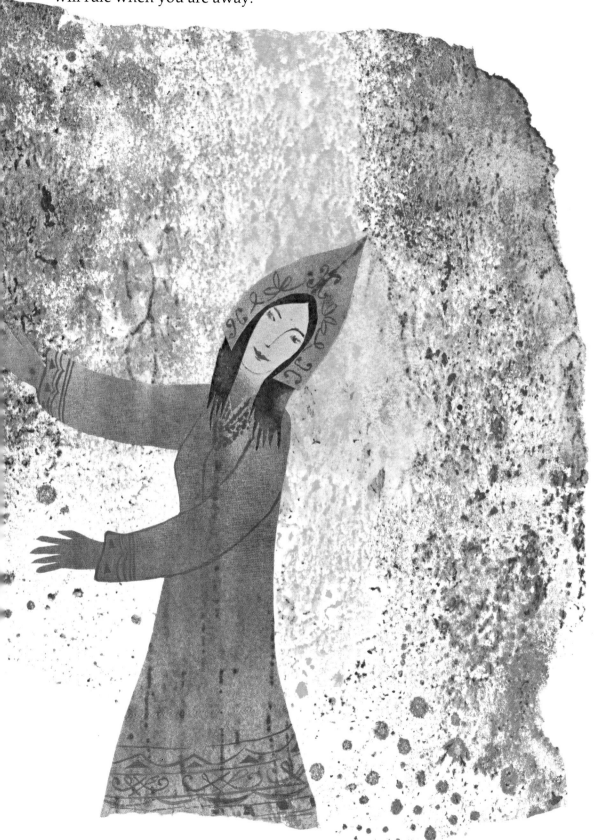

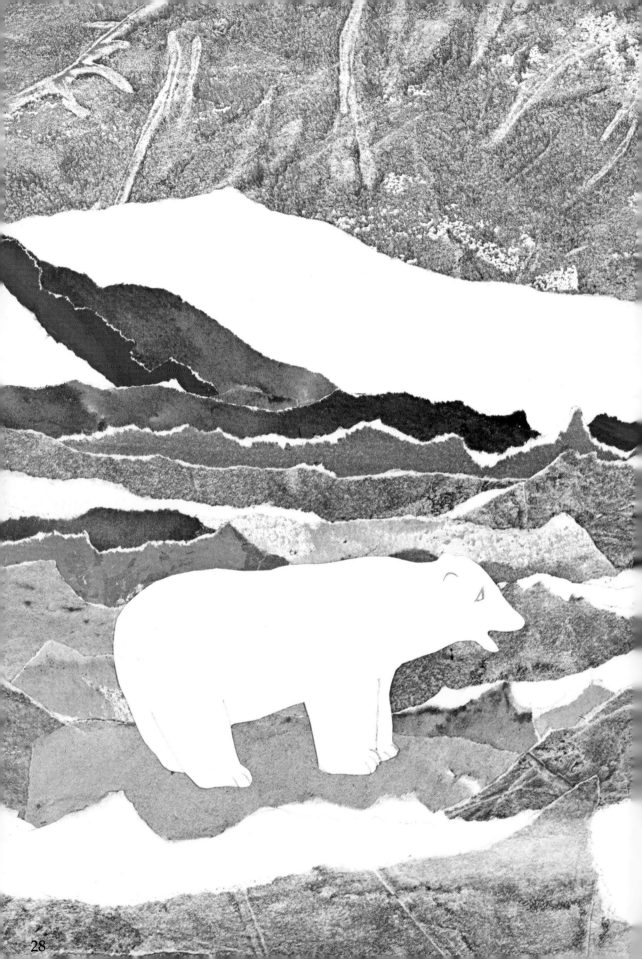

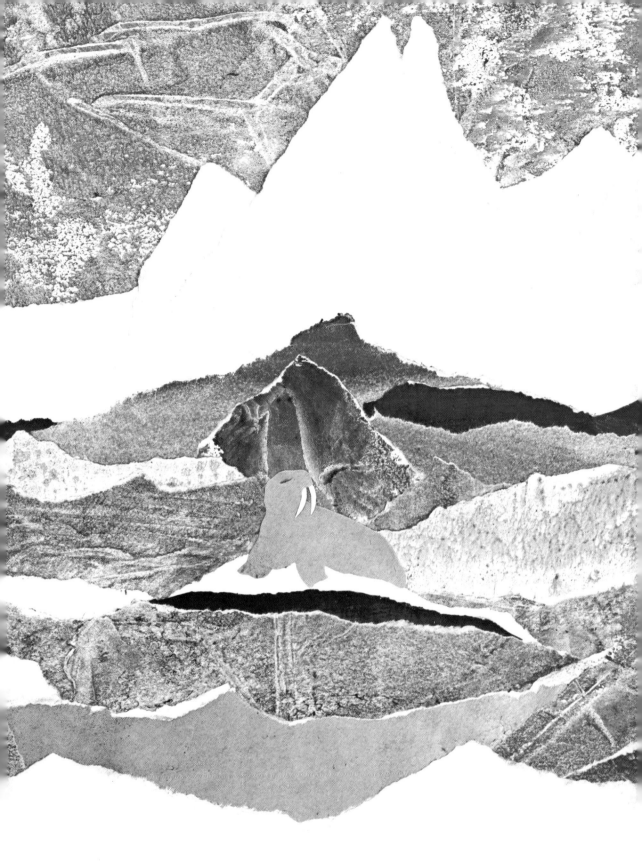

Winter could do nothing but agree to this. In the Far North he keeps the land in his strong and icy grip all year round. But he leaves in late autumn and comes back to Glooskap's country where he reigns for half the year.

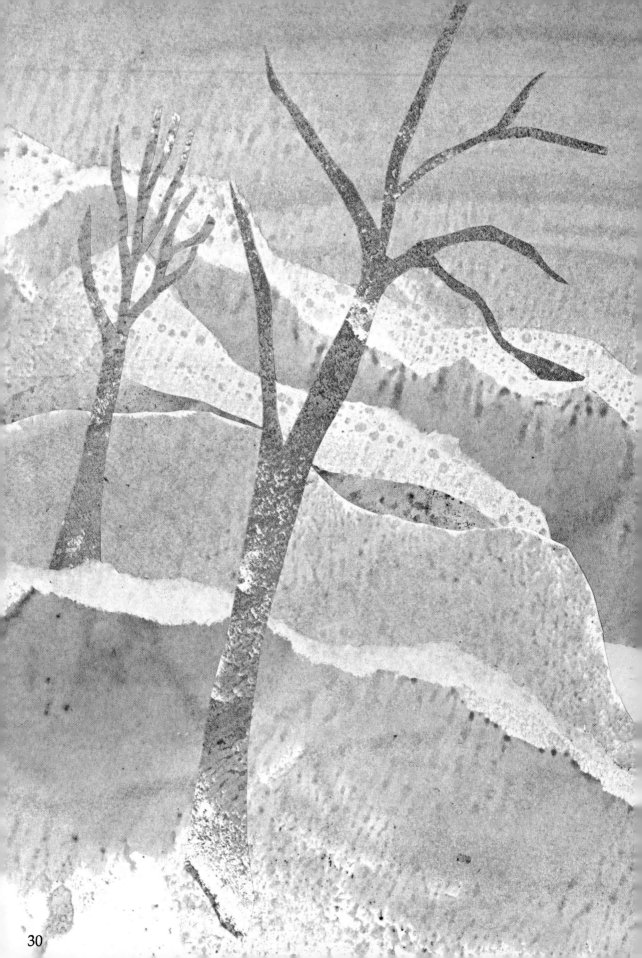

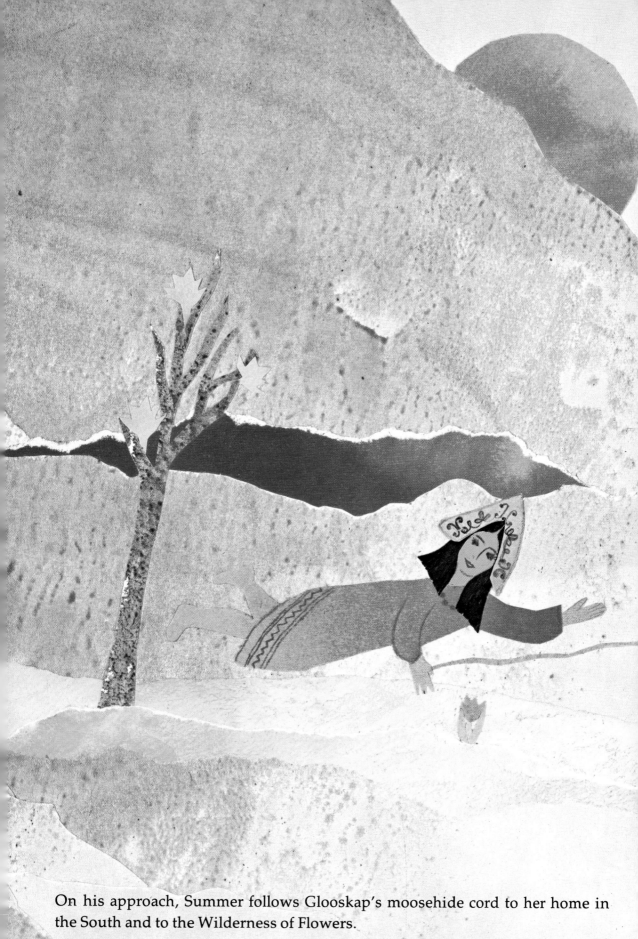

On his approach, Summer follows Glooskap's moosehide cord to her home in the South and to the Wilderness of Flowers.

But every year her love of Glooskap's country brings her back to awaken the earth from its deep sleep and bestow life on everything that grows. In this way Winter and Summer divide their rule between them in Glooskap's country.

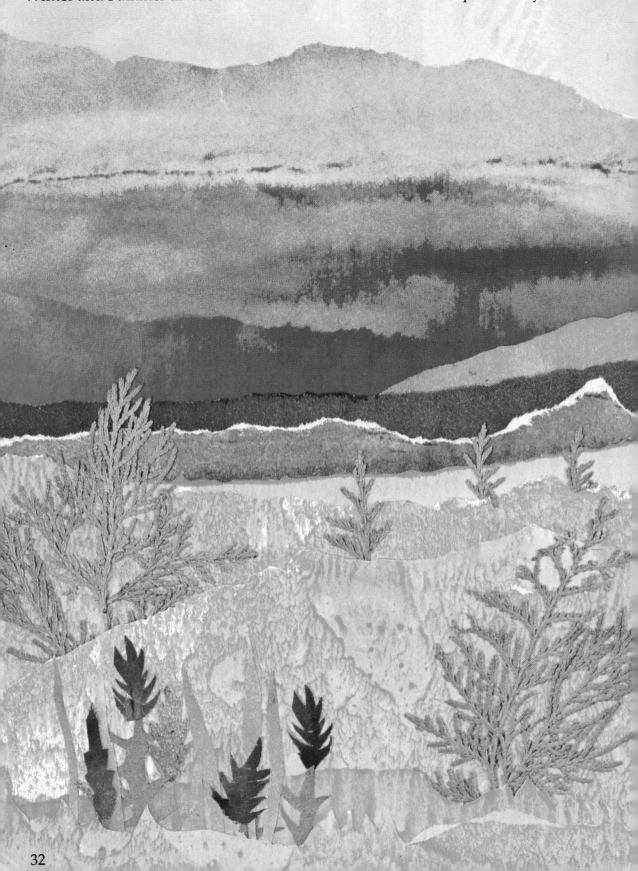